Lose the Excuses
and the Weight

LOSE THE EXCUSES AND THE WEIGHT

DARTANYAN ADKINS

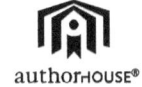

authorHOUSE®

AuthorHouse™
1663 Liberty Drive
Bloomington, IN 47403
www.authorhouse.com
Phone: 1-800-839-8640

First published by AuthorHouse   06/08/2011

ISBN: 978-1-4634-1102-2 (sc)
ISBN: 978-1-4634-1101-5 (ebk)

Library of Congress Control Number: 2011909805

Printed in the United States of America

Any people depicted in stock imagery provided by Thinkstock are models, and such images are being used for illustrative purposes only.
Certain stock imagery © Thinkstock.

This book is printed on acid-free paper.

Because of the dynamic nature of the Internet, any web addresses or links contained in this book may have changed since publication and may no longer be valid. The views expressed in this work are solely those of the author and do not necessarily reflect the views of the publisher, and the publisher hereby disclaims any responsibility for them.

INTRODUCTION

ALL MY LIFE, I've always been a big guy. Because of my size, my peers always laughed at me and picked on me. When I was in elementary school, I got into it with other classmates because they had a problem with something about me that I didn't understand then. I always thought to myself, *I don't bother or do anything to make them dislike me.* When I got older, it made sense to me. I was bigger than other peers my age. I had a combination of both fat and height. I must have weighed three hundred pounds then. I began to distance myself from all the others because I was tired of having to battle other kids my age because of my size. I began to hate school. I didn't want to go anymore because my size ashamed and embarrassed me. As I look back now, I wasn't big at all. I was just stocky for a kid my age, but I didn't have anyone telling me that. As I grew older and got further in elementary school, I stopped eating at school because I was ashamed to eat around other kids. I threw my body off. I skipped lunch and waited until I got home to eat. The human body has to get a certain amount of nutrition each day and consume at least three meals daily. Well, I stopped eating because I thought I was going to lose weight. As time went on and I acted like this every day at school, this made matters worse. As I got older, I became more isolated from my peers, and I led a more sedentary lifestyle. I got bigger and bigger. I'd eat and eat until I was full. I ate cakes, cookies, and those rolls with those special filling like apples and blueberries. I loved milk. I always told people I probably could have drank a whole cow filled with milk if I were thirsty enough. I loved milk, but not the 1 or 2 percent. Whole milk. I drank the shit out of some milk. My favorite nighttime snack was a quart of milk with a two-pound bag of baked beans. Yummy! That was the shit to me. Years of eating like that really added up, in weight that is.

Even crueler, it didn't stop there. It even followed me home. My father, a very foul, fucked-up individual, would talk about me to his friends and laugh with them about my size and how much I weighed. He'd tell them how big I was and tell them the size clothes I wore. I used to hate it, and it grew into a lot of hate and resentment toward my father. I always told my mom about how my dad and his friends poked and made fun of me. She'd always say, "He's just proud of you." But I knew that teasing with his friends wasn't pride or love. That spiraled my self-esteem into a downward plummet. I grew to hate him.As time went on and I grew older. and built a high self-esteem about myself, I bought larger clothes sizes and gained a bad attitude with it. I had no problem with being a big, heavy dude. Actually, I believe I was more confident and secure then than I am now, but my only problem was my clothes sizes.

Getting women wasn't a problem for me. I developed a cruel and harsh attitude when it came to women who didn't like me for me. My attitude was that, if a bitch didn't like me for me, then that was her loss. I knew I was and still am a kind, caring, affectionate man, so why should I waste my time on some senseless broad?

I hated and got tired of buying clothes that were only limited at a certain stores. I couldn't buy normal-sized T-shirts at places like Walmart or JCPennys. I had to go to a big-and-tall store and pay anywhere from twenty-five to fifty dollars for a T-shirt. My shorts, because that was all I wore, cost from fifty to sixty-five dollars a pair. I thought I'd never see a size fifty or fifty-four again in my life.

I decided I'd had enough. When I decided to make a life-altering change, my main goal was to just lose weight. At one doctor visit, I weighed myself, and I was shocked to find that I weighed five hundred and fifty pounds. That was enough to frighten me. I thought that, if I would have kept going on that way and kept getting bigger, I might have a stroke or massive heart attack one day and fall dead somewhere. That was my incentive to decide to make a big, life-alerting change. The gym I presently attend now was offering a special, six months for one hundred dollars. Soon after I heard about this membership offer, I hopped right on it. It was November 25, 2007. The gym called it a "Black Friday Special." I thought, *I'm jumping on this deal right away.* When I began working out, my only thought was, *The only way I'm going to lose this weight is to change my life completely. The only way to do this is to make a complete change of lifestyle, from the way I eat to the things I do on a day-to-day basis.* I didn't want to make it a temporary change, but a forever one. I wanted this life alteration a permanent one.

I knew the lifestyle I had wasn't working, so I wanted to try a different one. I didn't want to get involved with all those get-quick-fit weight loss programs. I always believed that, whatever you want, you have to work hard to get it. I felt those get-quick-fit options and surgeries were easy cop-outs and only for lazy people who were just looking for an easy way out. My philosophy is, "It wasn't quick putting it on, and it sure as hell isn't going to be quick taking it off. I" Also, not only are surgeries very expensive, they aren't guaranteed to work for everybody. A few people I know had the procedure done, and they didn't lose a single pound. To top it off, they still have to stick to a strict diet. Why waste your time and money and do all that hacking on your body when you can just follow some fundamental steps to do the same things I did? It doesn't cost you anything at all, and it's 100 percent guaranteed to work . . . well, as long you're willing to put in the effort.

Everybody is searching for that magical antidote—a wonder pill, program, or food—for weight loss. Millions of companies and marketers feed off people's laziness to sell their products for weight loss. The hard, solid truth is that there is none. Stop looking and praying for this miracle potion. You just have to get off your ass and put all that wishful thinking into motion. People are always asking me what I did, in reference to my weight loss. When I tell them, they say, "I tried. I can't." The way I see it, if they would put all that whining and negative thinking into energy and their muscles, maybe they might start noticing some positive results.

Like I mentioned earlier, everybody is looking for an easy way, but I'm sorry to inform you that there is none. So lose the excuses and the weight. From all my trials, errors, and experiments on altering my life, I have come up with three fundamentals I use today. I call them the three Cs: change, challenge, and consistent. You can utilize these basic steps with any exercise you perform. You need them to build or tone the body you have always dreamed of having.

In writing this book, I didn't want to make a long, winding, complex algebraic book on weight loss. Making a lifestyle change just requires a few basic guidelines, not solving a mathematical expression. Now, reading this book alone won't help you. This is a long-term commitment, and overnight results won't happen if you try these fundamentals once. These steps require time, patience, and true commitment. These, not some magic diet or pill, are the building blocks for building and creating the physique you have always wanted. These fundamentals are something you can use for the rest of your days. I feel these other exercise programs do work, but who is really going to jump up and down thirty to ninety minutes every day for the rest of his or her days to stay fit and healthy? Who is going to go mentally insane to get fit every day or kick in the air to stay flexible or limber? As we age, our body does, too, so can an elderly person go insane to get fit on a regular basis? Are your joints and legs ready for all that heavy pounding on hard concrete flooring. You must build and prep your body for all that heavy stomping and movements. Say you normally weighed one hundred and seventy to one hundred and seventy-five pounds in your life. You gained one hundred pounds in the last ten years. You started working out or bought on one of these group workout videos. Do you really think you or your body is going to withstand that kind of high aerobic dance rhythm? You might break a bone or tear a shin while doing it. You must start slow and build and tone your body first before you do that all-out dance shit. If you would use and adopt my fundamentals on altering your life, you will lose the excuses and the weight. I have been obese all my life, all through my teen and adult years. I didn't have any male role models in my life. Others picked on me. I got into fights. I made enemies because of my size. America frowns on fat. People ridicule and poke fun at fat people. People who hate or are disgusted by obesity find reasons to blame a person's medical condition on weight. You shouldn't give any attention or be bothered by these ignorant-ass people and their prejudice or let them stop you from doing whatever you want to do.

This is how ridiculous America is getting with obesity issues. Before my mother passed, a doctor told her that, if she didn't lose weight, she would have a massive heart attack. Years later, that same doctor died of cancer. Ironically, she outlived him, and she didn't die from a heart attack. Two years ago, I visited the doctor to have some skin tags removed. After he removed them, I asked what had caused them. He said it was because I was obese. I believed him because he was my doctor. Later in the conversation, he said that he himself had skin tags, and they were normal outbreaks on the body. I first thought, *He just told me that obesity was the reason for my skin tag*. Even people of medicine don't know shit and share the same prejudice, too, when it comes to overweight people. Everybody thinks fat is the number-one cause of every illness and disease that plagues America. In truth, fat affects people differently. I was five hundred and fifty pounds, and I never had high blood pressure or high cholesterol.

People of today are so uninformed about obesity that it has become a worldwide ignorance. If you feel you need to lose weight, then lose weight, but don't listen or allow someone else's prejudice to be the reason. You can't let people get to you about your size. How can you listen to a person who doesn't exercise or is genetically smaller himself or herself? We all have different biomechanics. Our bodies burn and store fat differently from person to person. One person can eat a pound of cake and burn it off faster than the next person could. So always keep in mind, the majority of the world's population discriminates against fat people. It's one of America's biggest prejudices. You should change for yourself and your health, not because of what the next person thinks or what society says about obesity. People will try to convince you and tell you anything to make you believe that your weight is the problem. Like I said, I have been obese all my life, and the only thing obesity did to me was shape and mold my personality. Obesity allowed me to understand the world and the people around me better.

Even science and medicine are confused about obesity. Some doctors say obesity is the cause for certain illnesses, like diabetes or high blood pressure; others doctors and researchers say some of these diseases are hereditary. These same people who do all these studies and lengthy research efforts can't pin where most of these diseases stem from. Diabetes and cancer are the two famous culprits. Some say fat has a chemical that causes the body to release a chemical that causes cancer, but a skinny man or woman who stays healthy and fit gets it. If obesity causes cancer and diabetes, then why does a person with a lower body mass index (BMI) get cancer? Stay clear of all these so-called studies and propaganda. Again, if your weight bothers you, then lose the shit. Don't do it on account of what other people and clinical studies say. You must decide to lose weight or change your life for yourself and not what science and medicine say. A doctor told my girlfriend, "You can't believe everything you read in these medical books."

CHANGE

W HEN I BEGAN my journey to a new life, I had no idea what I was going to do. I only knew one word, change. I knew I wanted to lose weight, and, to do this, I knew I had to change my whole life from the way I ate, the things I did on a daily basis, and, most importantly, the way I thought. You must understand that change must begin somewhere. It must start in the mind, the accelerator for change, first. When you recognize you need a change in your life, you have already made a step in applying the accelerator toward change.

I began with my intake, but I wasn't into counting calories. From experience, it's not how many calories you take in, but what is in there. I started with the foods I ate first. Now the key approach in changing up your foods is how you view the things you eat and drink. You see the better-selected food you choose as health foods or diet foods. If you look at the new choices in the food you eat as different or foods that normal people eat, it will be very difficult to stick to your new eating behavior. Now we are all familiar with the word "diet." The word "diet" gives off a restricting sound. It makes a person feel he or she will have to be committed to this certain way of eating in order to lose weight and get healthy, like he or she still can't enjoy the foods he or she always loved anymore, especially coming from an unhealthy, free-to-enjoy-whatever-kind-of-food-I-want lifestyle.

Don't use this word when you change your eating habits and start living healthy. It will only make you feel like you are in prison to this way of life, and you are not. Instead of using the word "diet," use the following words like alternate, different, better choice, or substitution. These words don't sound so imprisoning and restraining to the ear when used. You can even say, "I just choose to eat something more healthy" instead of saying, "I'm on a diet." Understand and realize that the changes in selecting the more nutritious foods are healthier alternatives than the ones that you and I grew up with. If I tell someone to go on a diet, he or she may frown at the idea because everyone has this conception that dieting consists of not eating the things you like or are used to eating, like cakes and cookies. But if I say, "Just substitute a piece of cake for one with fewer calories or eat cookies that are lower in sugar and fat," it doesn't sound as harsh as using the word "diet."

Remember, change starts in the mind first. I consume many fluids when I get thirsty, so I drink either low—or zero-calorie drinks. When you change your lifestyle, you don't have to worry about monitoring or being afraid of overdoing it because what you choose as a healthier alternative is not as bad for you compared to what you are used to eating or drinking. And it doesn't pack you down with loads of calories. So, like I mentioned previously, if I have a soft drink or any type of juice, I have one with few or no calories. Many people told me that they hate the taste of diet drinks because they don't taste the same as normal soft drinks. Or some will say, "You can drink one, but don't drink a lot of them." Regular soft drinks are loaded with tons of calories and sugar. Sugar then turns into more calories, effectively packing on the pounds. If you are sincere about changing the way you look and getting healthy, you must adjust what you eat and the way you view the things you eat. If you cannot bear drinking diet drinks, try reduced-calorie soft drinks. They are healthy and reduced in calories.

The last tip to remember is reduction. When you decide to have a healthier lifestyle, you look for the same foods you normally eat, but in a reduced form. Like I mentioned previously about having the cookies, have them in a reduced version. For example, if you drink whole milk, try 2 percent. If you can stand drinking skim milk (0 percent fat), then make a switch to that version instead. See, you didn't stop drinking milk overall, but you chose a better and healthier choice. The lower percent of fat content is always better and healthier. The less fat you have in your selection of food choices, the better you will be, and the healthier you will become.

Again, not only does change modify how and what you eat, it works on how you think. You must think and know that the change you make is a change for the best for you and your loved ones. And in order to remain healthy and fit after you made these adjustments, you must stay at it and make this a lifelong journey. Changing your eating behavior for short lengths of time and returning to your old behaviors will only cause you pain and disappointment. You have to be fed up and decide to tell yourself, "This is a change forever." You must have a reason to change your life, for example, your health, being around to see your child or children grow up, or just wanting to look and feel better.

Fear and wanting to fit in normal-sized clothes motivated me. I was sick and tired of having to buy large sizes and then paying higher prices because of that. I always had big legs and carried most of my weight in my thighs, so, when I couldn't buy normal fitted pants that were a certain cut, I had to buy bigger-than-normal-sized pants or a short size to compensate for my legs. I was paying a lot more money for clothes than a smaller man would. I had a fairly decent waist size, but my huge thighs made it impossible to purchase smaller pants or shorts. I could have fit in a waist size of fifty-eight or sixty, but I had to buy a size seventy. I was so fed up with dealing with these issues that most people never think about. I decided I'd had enough. That is why I say you must initiate change in your mind. I believe in taking baby steps, not large leaps toward weight loss success. Large leaps only lead one into larger disappointments and upsets. So when I speak of change, I'm talking about mentality, not just activities and food. Like I said, you must change all aspects of your life if you expect to get fit and healthy.

I know how it is, not knowing where and when to start. I started out at five hundred and fifty pounds, and I didn't have a clue about how to begin losing weight and getting healthy. You must begin a little bit at a time, and I suggest you first start with what you eat. Learn how to select healthier foods, that is, foods lower in sugars, calories, fats, and, if you do have high blood pressure, cholesterol. If you eat large portion sizes at meals, eat the same portion, but in reduced versions. You can't cut your meal sizes into smaller portions until you learn how to adapt to your new eating behavior. If you try cutting your meal portions down cold turkey before you practice how to make healthier food selections, you will only run a high chance of relapsing back to your old eating habits and wasting all that time. I'm trying to teach you and show you how to eat the same foods in a healthier and slower manner. Don't try to dive right in to eating healthy. Slowly and gradually make changes to your food selection. Carefully pick your food. Read the nutrient label very carefully. Compare brand name to store brands because some brands are healthier than others are. I found most store brands are more nutritious than popular name brands and cost less. Create an eye for super foods, that is, foods high in the good stuff (vitamins, minerals, and protein) and low in the bad stuff (fat, trans fat, saturated fat, and cholesterol). Remember, you didn't get unhealthy overnight, so you will not get healthy in a day. You must train yourself how to eat right, stamp eating and being healthy in your head, and always be on the lookout for healthier food choices.

This is a long process itself and can take years to master. Portioning your food sizes is not as effective as selecting the type of foods you consume. For example, compared to an apple, you can get more calories and sugar out of a small piece of cake. If you enjoy frequent snacking, it's a whole lot healthier to eat a pear with a glass of Crystal Light than a piece of cake with a glass of whole milk.

Now you do have some foods you must cut out period. Cakes and pies are simply not good to consume at all. They offer no kind of nutritious value at all, and they are loaded with calories, fat, and sugars. In comparison, you have many more healthy foods to choose from. For me, I eat tons of fruit and nuts. I personally love trail mixes, and it gets me very full with a few glasses of non-caloric soft drinks or water. Trail mixes can be used as a dessert or a midday meal. I use them for both. Trail mixes gives you the benefit of both worlds. You get the nuts and dry fruits all in one package, along with high nutrients that the two have. If you are going to use trail mixes as your alternative, purchase the trail mix with the nuts and the dry fruits, not the ones with the candy-coated nuts.

If you aren't a big fruit eater, try dehydrated fruits. They make an excellent choice for snacking. Dehydrated fruits are very healthy, and you can keep them in your refrigerator for a long time. Another great snack to choice from is pretzels, and they can be used as a midday meal or a snack. Pretzels have no fat, and they are very low in calories. Stay away from the pretzels with all the special coated flavorings and seasonings. Use only the sourdough kind. Washed down with a few glasses of non-caloric soft drinks, pretzels make a great alternative food choice.

My advice is to not limit yourself on fruits and nuts. Eat as much as you like. Fruits and nuts are very healthy, and they are complex carbs so they digest very slowly and will not pack on as many sugars and calories as cakes and cookies.

Over the years, I personally haven't changed how much I ate. I changed what I ate instead. I have always been a big eater, so, when I changed my eating behavior, I learned it wasn't the size of the plate, but what was on the plate. So don't change your portion sizes; adjust what you are eating and its nutritional content. Try eating a pound of apples compared to a pound of cake. Your stomach can't tell if it has sixteen ounces of fruit inside of it compared to a twelve-ounce piece of cake, but your body will process the two totally differently. And you will see it when you get on the scale. You must make better decisions on what you eat, not necessarily the portion size. Plus, if you want to lose weight and get healthy, you must change the way you live and eat. You can't lose weight and remain eating the same. You must change if you want to see a difference. Your body will automatically begin to eat at the fat when you start making these small adjustments because you're not feeding it what it has been used to eating for all these years. If you are a heavyset person, reducing your caloric intake by the choices you make in the food you eat will certainly cause your body to start eating away at the fat. Trust and believe me. Portion size is not always key when it comes to trimming down.

In today's society, I know we are all busy and don't really have time to sit down for a home-cooked meal. Everybody wants a meal right away, which made places like McDonald's and Jack in the Box the number-one places to go to eat. Eating out is okay, but where you eat is the problem. A double cheeseburger with fries has whole lot more calories than a few pieces of grilled chicken with sides of pinto beans and two pieces of corn on the cob. Can you see the difference in the selection of meals and the healthier choices? Eating out is not bad as long as you make healthier selections. I love grilled chicken, so, if I'm dining out, I'd go to this restaurant called El Pollo Loco, a very famous restaurant in California. I have a four-piece meal, chicken with two sides of pinto beans. It sounds plain and not fulfilling, but it's a great meal. It's somewhat costly, but the price to get and stay healthy is very well worth it. If you don't like the menu selection, you can have the BRC burrito, but no cheese, please. Cheese isn't good for you, and it's loaded with lots of carbs and fat. Another great alternative for dining out is KFC. Years back, KFC was a place you stayed away from as well, but now they have added the grilled chicken, a healthier menu selection. Their grilled chicken is very delicious, and it's grilled and seasoned very well. Price is the only drawback to eating at KFC. Again, healthy eating comes with a price. But if you choose to eat there, just have the grilled chicken and the corn on the cob or the beans. It's not how much you eat, but what you eat.

Now if you like buffet dinning, that's great, but make sure you eat the lean meats and vegetables. Stay away from the battered food because it's not good and very unhealthy. Fried whatever is a sure enough way to pack on the unwanted calories and cholesterol. Battered anything is always filled with trans fat and fat. Battered food clogs your heart and arteries. If you are going to eat at a buffet, select meats that are lean in fats, such as chicken that has been grilled or boiled. Grilled anything is an absolute plus, because all the fat and skin has been burnt off. Now beef is okay, but make sure it's lean. I suggest you stay completely away from ground beef because it's loaded with tons of calories and fat. If you are a big meat eater like myself, try ground turkey. My beautiful girlfriend turned me on to ground turkey years ago, and it's the best thing that has happened to my health and me since prison. Ground turkey is a thousand times healthier than ground beef, and it has a very low fat content. It's back to what I stated previously about making healthier selections. When cooked, ground turkey tastes just the same as ground beef, if not better. So if you decide to use ground turkey as one of your select poultries, use it as all your main meat dishes.

If you want to lose weight and get healthy, you must change. You can't sit on your ass and whine and pout about how much you need to lose the weight. You can't use your medical situation or work as an excuse for why you can't get healthy. You must take small steps. Start making little adjustments in your life every day. Just starting by changing your food intake will bring you change. You don't have starve yourself to lose weight, but make healthier selections in what you take in every day. If you can't get to the gym every day, try once or twice a week. Once you learn how to use this fundamental step, little by little, you will lose the excuses and the weight.

CHALLENGE

FORGET ABOUT THOSE outdoor places to exercise that some claim to save you tons of dollars like walking in the local parks, jogging around your neighborhood, or placing an exercise machine in your garage. Save your money and time. Exercising at your home, local parks, or any other place other than the gym will only distract you from your workout. For example, a friend may come over, your child may need you, or a friend or relative may call you with an important message. You need to be in a place where you are totally separated from everything and everybody that involves you. You need to be in a place where you are completely isolated from the world so you can focus on you and your exercise. In the gym, you aren't distracted or disturbed. You can't just stop and go do something and start working out again. Constantly doing this stop-and-go workout won't help you to build up your endurance level. Being in the gym keeps you focused and concentrated on your routine and allows you to receive full maximum effort. Many trainers (or so-called trainers) say mix it up and do some cardio with some free weights. Forget about it. I recommend you begin with cardio first. Why? You want to:

- Do lots of experimenting before you start taking on a program that requires you to incorporate doing weight training and cardio
- Learn how to get into the groove of one type of exercise
- See what does and doesn't work for you

You can do both cardio and weight training, but, if have been sitting on your ass for years, that is a lot of work on your body and mind. Before you start taking on cardio and weight training, you need to find something you enjoy and is relaxing and easy for you and your body. In this chapter, I will:

- Define challenge
- Explain how to challenge yourself
- Detail the importance of challenging self
- Explain step-by-step the things you must do in order to conquer the challenges you set out for yourself

First, you must start at exercising slow, not in terms of speed, but beginning slow. You can't rush headfirst into losing weight and trying to lose tons of weight. Rushing and trying to get fit quickly will only lead to disappointment if you don't see results. I have seen many people who enter the gym for their first month and attend almost every day, and, when a few months go by, I don't see them anymore. Again, you didn't get the size you are overnight, so taking it off will not come quickly either. You want to find what is comfortable for you and an exercise you enjoy doing. This is key, and it's going to be your bread and butter if you expect to see lasting major results in the gym. Cardio training is easier to start out because you can do as much as your body can stand and stop when you feel fatigued. Weight training puts more demand on your body. So again, if you are just beginning, start with cardio and find what works best for your body. Stay with it for a while or until you have lost the body weight you wanted and you feel a need to tone up.

When searching for exercise or machine type, you want to find an exercise that you like and is comfortable for you. This is very important because, if you don't like a certain type of exercise, you won't stay on it every day, and you will be less productive on it. This is just like doing something you like doing all the time. If you like doing something or have a passion for it, your mind will be focused on the thing you enjoy. Cardio is demanding on the body, so you want to be okay with the exercise and machine of your choice. You want to get familiar with the machine you choose and allow your body to get the feel (how your body moves and respond to the machine) of the machine, too. When using any cardio machine, you should look for the machine's mechanism functions for example, the machine's smoothness (how your foot strikes the machine pad, like a treadmill, or the ease of how your leg rotates on a bike or elliptical machine). Does the machine turn easily, or is it very hard? You don't want the machine to suddenly slip when you are in the middle of an exercise. A cardio machine should be a smooth, tight flow of speed, not too easy or too hard to use.

Doing any cardio machine will cause other parts of your body to work, so you need to work out on the machine of your choice long enough to build up those other body parts. You want to give your body time to loosen up on the machine. This is another reason why sticking to one machine is beneficial. Compared to just sticking to one exercise all the time, circuit training doesn't bring these type of benefits. It may take you months or even a year to build up these other body parts. Again, time will bring you there. Just stay consistent with your routine. If you don't already have a particular machine or exercise you like, experiment with different kinds that your gyms offers. Again, find a machine you are very comfortable exercising on. Once you find a machine you like, just begin working out a little bit at a time. When I say "a little bit," I mean you do much as you can do or until you start getting that huffing-and-puffing breathing. For example, if your machine of choice is the bike, start out doing five or ten minutes on it. Don't try to go hours at a time at it because you must allow your body to build and strengthen itself first and you don't want to be mentally burnt out.

For the latter, your mind will register this as how it is going to feel whenever you work out, so, on the days you don't feel so cranked up to exercise, your mind has a negative impression on moving your body. So don't put that impression in your head. You want to be eager and self-driven to work out every time you begin your time in the gym. You want a feeling of discontentment from your last workout, like you must work out because you didn't give it your all the last time. You think you could have done more the last time, so you're going to push it even further. This is the element of challenge. If you feel like that wasn't challenging enough, bump up the machine in small increments, like fifteen or twenty minutes. Once you start feeling fatigue or reach that huffing-and-puffing breathing, stop and end your workout for the day. You don't want to overexert yourself the first day or week. Again, you will only burn yourself out fast. You want to push yourself little by little, but not in one session. You want do enough to just get a rapid heartbeat or the huffing and puffing going. Once you start building up your stamina and feel like twenty to thirty minutes isn't enough to work out, then you may want to work out for longer periods of time. You have built your heart and lungs in order to build up your endurance and stamina. You must first learn how to enjoy and be comfortable doing your workout routine before you try being in the gym for long periods of time.

Before you begin your workout program, set a goal for yourself and work toward that aim. Setting a goal in your workout is another key element for weight loss and getting healthy and fit. Here is what I mean. If your goal is running a mile and you can't run a quarter mile, then, every time you work out, aim to reach that mile. Now when you start running and you start breathing hard when you are around a tenth of a mile, this is what I call the "red zone." Like a red zone in a car that tells the driver how hard the car is working, this is the body's red zone. This is where your heart really starts pumping and lungs start inhaling and exhaling air. Once you find your red zone or fatiguing mark in the gym, you always want to work out around or in this zone. The longer and more often you work out doing this kind of heavy breathing, you are building your heart and lungs. Working in or around your red zone is how you build a strong, more efficient cardiovascular system. In this zone, you start really burning calories and melting the fat. Exercising in or around your red zone is key to building up your endurance and stamina. Every time you begin your workout routine, you challenge yourself to get to your destination or goal. You aim to reach your point and work in your red zone as long as you possibly can. Working out like this will build your cardiovascular fast. So if you set out to run, walk, or jog a mile and you start getting in your red zone around the quarter mile mark, you keep on until you can't bear running any farther. The next time you work out, you do the same, but you push it a little farther than you did the last time. Every time you are in your red zone, you tell yourself, "I will go a little more." You keep on, no matter how hard you are breathing. This is what I mean in challenging yourself. You set a goal or point to reach, and you work toward your aim every time you work out. When you come near or closer than you were the previous workouts, you tell yourself, "I will go a little farther this time."

Gauging or metering your workout is also another helpful practice in the gym. Some people gauge their workout in different ways. Some people use minutes; others, like myself, use miles. This is a matter of personal preference. I like going by miles. For example, if I felt I have built the endurance to do a mile with ease or it is no longer hard for me anymore, I work toward going for another mile. I like ending my workouts at equal numbers. For example, if I knock out one mile on the treadmill, my next goal is to reach my second mile, not that same day, but every time I work out. So again, I work out until I'm near or close to my second mile. I do this every day or however long it takes me to complete my mission. Once I have completed my second mile, I end my workout. I feel I have completed my mission that day. I don't try to take on another mile after just finishing my second mile. I'm not trying to burn myself out. Again, you don't want to tear yourself down or go on an exercising binge because you feel your level of cardio has increased. I know I sometimes get that kind of feeling, but I save it for the next scheduled workout day. Just do enough to keep the burning desire red-hot. I keep doing this for weeks or months until doing two miles or whatever is easy to do. I continue using this same approach whenever I feel I have built up the endurance where I feel I can do my third or fourth mile. You can use this type of training approach in any exercise you choose. Subconsciously, you are challenging yourself. You are setting a goal in your mind and aiming to defeat that objective. This fundamental will bring you great endurance and strength. When I began my workout, I didn't want anyone to help me lose weight. My goal was to lose weight, and that was all. I wasn't really concerned about how long it took me to do it. I just wanted to lose weight and get healthy for the rest of my life. I told one of the personnel who signed me in the gym, "I don't want a trainer or anybody helping me." I wanted to do this all by myself. I know how these gyms work, and I know these so-called trainers are not in it to better me or anybody else

Using this basic step in your new workout regime, you don't need a trainer, or "bank-robbing trainers," as I call them. Some say they can help you lose weight and eat healthy. Yeah, if you use those guys for a month, you'll be exercising at the homeless shelter. Those guys aren't in the business to help you lose weight and stay healthy and fit. They are a bunch of idiots who can't get their own health life right. They don't know shit about weight loss. The gym officials only hired them to help put money in the gym's bank account. These so-called trainers are small, skinny men and women who are naturally thin. Sure, they can tell you how and what to eat because you look at them and think, "This is what they do to stay the size they are." Sorry, they do not eat healthy at all. They never had to go through trying to shed weight or make alterations to lose weight and stay healthy. They don't have to, nor do they share the same problematic issues as you. Most smoke and drink. Most importantly, they have little or no education about sports nutrients and health. They are just trying to earn a commission off the money you pay to have a personal trainer. They use your insecurity and laziness to feed their family and keep their job, and that's it. So stay clear of those guys, and save your time and hard-earned dollars. Remember this, you put the weight on, so you are going to have to take it off.

Challenging is a preset goal you put in your mind to seek out to conquer. I believe that, when you set a goal to do anything in your life, no matter what it is, you challenge yourself to get to your aim. In this context, challenging yourself to reach a certain distance or time every time you work out. You tell yourself, "I will get there, no matter what it takes." Subconsciously, we do that when we set a goal for ourselves and aim toward it. We are challenging ourselves. You say, "I want that, whatever it is, so I'm going to do whatever it takes to get it." Don't worry if you didn't achieve your goal the first time. Every day or every other day, just keep telling yourself that you will push it a little further. Before you even realize it, you have conquered your goal. In a sense, it's determination on steroids. When you set a challenge for yourself, you don't think about how long it will take to reach your goal or, in this case, mark. You just head toward it until you reach it. You don't let anything distract you from heading there. You bang at it hard to break down those barriers standing in your way. You say, "I want it!" And you set your mind toward getting it. That is how you must think when you challenge yourself. If you don't think like that, then you will never lose the weight and be healthy. When things that try to stop you from getting to your mark (people, life issues, and, most importantly, pain) pressured you, you tell yourself, "I can do it!" And you keep pressing until you hit your mark. That is the attitude you must have when you challenge yourself. So if you are breathing hard as hell and your goal is to run or walk a mile and you are three-quarters away, you tell yourself, "I'm going to make this mile." And you push until you get there I have always kept in my mind and said to myself when I first began, "I will start out a little bit at a time." I wasn't trying to lose a huge amount of weight all at once because, realistically, I knew that was impossible to do. I knew it was going to take me a while, so I decided to just take it slow, day by day. Like I said, I wanted to make this a forever change for the rest of my life. I wanted to live and breathe. I wanted to get fit and healthy and stay that way forever. I wanted to make the gym my second home. I wanted exercising to come second nature in my life, just like when I sat around and did nothing but eat up everything except the kitchen sink. It was second nature for me to eat all kinds of different things, so I knew eating right and staying healthy was doing the same thing. Sitting on your ass and devouring a box of cookies is a habitual behavior, but so is eating right and getting fit. You must make it habitual. I didn't want to play the yo-yo game, that is, lose a few pounds and gain it back and more. I wanted the weight off and to keep it off for good. I believe one should have this kind of thinking. I feel you shouldn't try to rush getting fit. Take your time, and work at it every day. Make it a habit that you do every day all day. Getting and staying active every day will bring results. You have to work steadily and have patience.

Years before, I was a member at another gym. Back then, I enjoyed using the recumbent bike to do cardio. So when I signed with the gym I'm in today, that's all I did. I started out doing just one mile on the bike. (I gauge my workout by mile per hour.) I'd normally work around speeds of six mile per hour and keep at that pace for five miles on the bike. At that rate of speed, I can really start feeling my body work. My heart starts pumping, and my lungs really start puffing and sucking in air. So when I found a pace I was okay doing and a point I wanted to reach, I made that my mark to reach every time I began working out. I set in my mind that was going to be my goal to reach—or wanted to reach—every time I started my workout. Every time I began my workout, I started exercising at that speed and worked up to that distance. In my mind, I set that as my goal every time I worked out to hit that five-mile distance. Throughout time, I had built the stamina to go farther, so I made in my mind to go to six miles. This is where I began to understand all I was doing was challenging myself. When fatigue kicked in, I told myself, "I'm going to push it a little more." That is how you challenge yourself. Just find a machine you are comfortable on and enjoy exercising on, set a point or destination in your mind that you plan to—or want to—reach every time you work out, and aim to reach toward that point (or "mark") every time nonstop.

When you begin your change of life (or life-altering lifestyle), I don't like using the word "diet." You may need to do a little experimenting. So if you join a gym and you don't have a clue what exercises to do, try them all. You can really only choose from three. The exercise machine that works best is totally personal preference. I personally enjoy the treadmill and bike. I now use the treadmill as my main cardio machine. Some like the elliptical machine over the treadmill; others say the stair-climber is great. I say try whatever works best and gets your heart pumping.

Like I said previously, I don't suggest or recommend circuit training at all. I get tired of hearing trainers telling people circuit training is best to shock the body and to switch up the exercise. Once again, you can't listen to a bunch of guys who only care about keeping their job and getting a commission check, which I think is around 5 to 10 percent of your hard-earned money. I'm not a really big advocate of circuit training. Depending on one's body, it takes thirty to forty-five minutes to get the body fully warmed up. Circuit training doesn't give the body enough time to warm up thoroughly enough. You must learn how to get a feel of the machine because each is different. You don't want to just hop on and then hop off. You must teach your body how to really learn how to get the feel of the machine and build a systematic rhythm on it. Don't worry about major weight loss. Again, that will come when you learn how to use and work the machine of your choice. Circuit training doesn't allow that because you aren't focusing on the workout and pacing, but getting to the next machine. You can't develop a groove or smooth pace for yourself because you aren't on the machine long enough. You need to teach yourself how to focus just solely on one machine. Focusing on one machine and keeping a steady pace will cause your body to start heating up and burning calories. Now you don't have to spend hours and hours on the machine of your choice, just enough time to get that huffing-and-puffing breathing or a heavy breath going. You don't want to burn yourself out or try to be like the person next to you who just ran six miles at seven to eight miles an hour. Believe me, if you keep reading and following my advice from this book, your level of endurance will skyrocket in no time. Oh, yeah, just to add, the person who ran six to seven miles has probably been doing that for years and has the body and lungs to do that kind of running. You, on the other hand, may have to work at it a little bit. So don't worry about getting to that level. Just focus on learning how to work out efficiently and effectively. So again, leave circuit training alone. Focus on the machine you like; perfect it pace by pace or minute by minute. This is where you challenge yourself and your body.

You don't have to push yourself every time you work out. You do have to keep pushing yourself every other day or time to time. Squeezing a little more out of your workout is going to build that endurance and increase your stamina. So every time you get around or near that mark and you are in your red zone, you are building your heart and lungs, not just your body. So the challenge you give yourself benefits you in all parts of your body. Once you have learned how to challenge and get in tune with your workout, you can ease off a little bit. Give yourself a break for hitting your workouts hard. You don't want to bang at your workout hard every day because you will wear out your body. For example, when I complete my first challenge or goal, I say to myself, "I'm not going to hit it hard today." I may do, let's say, a mile, but with a little intensity added. Here I can either challenge myself to another mile or stay at a mile but with little added intensity. I'm still exercising, keeping my body fit, staying active, and burning fat, but not working out as hard. You don't have to kill yourself every time you hit the gym. You don't want to torture your body like that because you may get burnt out or feel like the gym is torturing you. That will only leave you with desires of not wanting to return. You want to have a burning desire to return to the gym. So when you have achieved your goal and feel you have built the endurance, you can continue doing your mile or whatever your goal was, but add a little more intensity to your workout. Here's how you can do that. If your goal is running a mile and you bust your ass for months and months and finally reach running a mile, you run the same mile, but, this time, you incline the treadmill or run up a steep hill, wherever you choose to work out. If you run a mile in ten minutes, you run it harder and aim for eight or nine minutes. Once again, you challenge yourself to set out to push yourself to reach that eight, nine, or whatever minutes you choose to do your mile in. You never want to keep running the same mile at the same pace, especially if the mile comes with ease at doing. You have to switch it up a little and add a little more intensity. This will bring shock to the body, which will also build your endurance level even more. So if your goal is a mile with added intensity and you feel the pain or fatigue start kicking in, don't stop until you finish your mile.

At times, you will get bored doing the same repetitive routine. We all get that feeling from time to time. At times, you will not be in the mind-set or feel motivated to go all out or bang hard at your workout. You may have financial problems or something in your life that is bothering so much that you just don't feel like being in the gym. I know how this feels. I work out five days a week a week for ninety minutes each time, sometimes less than that. Again, I don't suggest hitting the gym that hard unless you really have the drive and endurance to spend that kind of time working out in the gym. Just do enough to get you a hard breath from your workout and leave immediately. Don't try to be a gym super athlete or show-off. You are there to get healthy and fit, not show the next man how long you can stay in the gym working out. If you're a man, leave the male ego shit at the house or in the bar with your pals. This is a lifelong commitment, not a month of show-and-tell. You are committing yourself forever and aiming to unearth and chisel the type of body you have always dreamed of having, so it's going to take time to do this. Building a body like this doesn't come cheap or overnight.

Like I stated earlier, you will get burnt out or unmotivated to hit the gym hard at times. When you get these types of feelings, do the following. Before you get ready to head in the gym, isolate yourself for a while. Don't place your mind on working out. Sit in your car (or wherever you are) and relax for a few, rather it be ten or thirty minutes. Sit somewhere by yourself, and somewhat unwind and put yourself in a complete solitude state of mind. Listen to some music or give someone a call. The point is to take your mind off the gym and not think about working out. Just relax yourself, take your mind off working out, and place it on other things. If you are having personal problems, think about and figure out how you are going to handle them. Try to solve them before you head in the gym. Some may say you should do the opposite, but working out while thinking about your problem will only make your workout boring and hard to get into. You need to clear your thoughts and free your mind before you head into the gym. We all have personal issues that trouble us, but you need to leave all your problems and worries somewhere else other than the gym. You may want to sit in your car and close your eyes for a while. Give yourself some "me time" before you go in. Again, take a few minutes and leave your problems outside the gym. Get your body and mind prepared to blast hard at your workout.

When you are finished and ready to enter the gym, don't just hit the machine hard. You're human, and those thoughts or worries might not leave you so soon. Start out slow or at a slower pace than you normally do. This speed allows you to still think about whatever you have on your mind without focusing too much on your workout just yet. Now you want to gradually start picking up the speed or pace on your machine. Here, you will start allowing your mind to shift to your workout. Just remember to start out slow and concentrate in your head. Start moving your mind from your problems to your workout at hand. You don't want to think about your problems, but I know it's hard to get into the rhythm when something bothers me. Before you know it, the feelings that cause you to feel down, worried, unmotivated, or bored will soon go away. That's why I tell people that they should warm up first before starting to work out. Warming up is a pre-workout for the mind and body.

You may feel sick while you are in the gym. Flu season or change of weather can affect your body and how you feel physically. If you feel ill or sick and don't feel like hitting the gym, go anyway, but don't hit it so hard when you work out. Bring yourself up to your normal speed, but don't add any kind of resistance. When you will feel achy and weak, you don't want to push yourself hard. Just move enough to get the blood flowing and your body warmed up. When exercising being sick and weak, your body will work extra harder than normal because of the viral infection your body is already trying to fight off. When you are sick and you work out, your body will sweat more, which is good because you're forcing your body to push harder. That helps rid you of all those infected blood cells and helps the body produce new cells. After a long, hard drive in the gym, you should load up on medicine and take tons of vitamin C. Take a long, hot, steamy shower, and get plenty of sleep. There is nothing better for the body after it has been physically stressed than a long period of sleep and rest. Once you get past your sick day, you will feel fresh and brand-new again. Don't let being sick stop you from working out. Just ease off the accelerator a little.

Now feeling tired and drowsy is very hard to manage or shake off. Not getting enough sleep the night before is hell on your body the next day, especially when it comes to working out. Getting plenty of sleep is key to a good workout. The body must receive at least seven to eight hours of sleep. Sleep is key for healing, recovery, and the body's metabolism. If you didn't get enough sleep for some reason and you feel tired but don't want to skip a day's workout, again, just take it slow on the machine. Don't blast right into your workout. Your body needs to begin cycling blood flow and get your blood sugar low to begin burning fat instead of muscle.

Physical pain will also make you not want to hit the gym. When you begin working out in the first few months, your body will go through a few days of aches and pain. Coming from a sedentary kind of lifestyle and switching to a more active one, your body won't be used to this strenuous type of stress. Figuratively speaking, your body will be screaming at you from all angles. Your legs may shout at you from time to time. Your back may tell you it's tapping out. Your arms may tell you they've had enough. Your body isn't used to this kind of strenuous activity. You must allow your body to adapt to these changes naturally. You will experience all kinds of muscle aches and pain all over your body. If running is your exercise of choice, you will experience knee, shin, calves, ass, or glute pain. All these muscles may even ache all at once. Don't panic or rush to the hospital. Normal body pain comes with daily exercise. For months, I was experiencing shin pain in both my legs from just power walking. Stretching is a great remedy to help ease the pain because it helps alleviate your body's aches and pain. Stretching the muscles allows the muscle to let blood flow easily and loosen up the muscle tissue. If you are preparing to do any type of exercise, it's best to stretch your entire body. Here's my advice before you begin your workout. Take five to ten minutes stretching the body part you are about to use in your workout. You don't have to spend a thousand hours stretching. Just spend enough time to get that loose feeling in your muscles. It also helps to stretch other muscles that you will be using in conjunction with the body part you will be using the most. For example, if you plan to run, not only do you want to stretch your quadriceps muscles, but you want to stretch your calves, glutes, and hamstrings as well. All these muscles work together in making the ability to run. So get a full body warm-up and stretch before you begin any vigorous workout for long lengths of time.

Finally, foot pain is another type of pain that doesn't just go away in a matter of days, especially if you are heavyset person and not used to being on your foot actively for a length of time. Again, you must learn how to stretch and warm up your foot like any other muscle in your body. Now foot pain also originates from bad or improper footwear. I have further details on using and having proper gym wear in the next chapter.

You don't want to be sick or anything else to stop you from getting healthy and fit. Allowing anything to disrupt you from your routine throws you off and keeps you from achieving your ultimate goal. Also, using these as reason to not work out only turns into excuses. Sure, I was sick, and I didn't feel up to work out some days, but I decided that this was going to be my life. That belief got me to the size I am today. I started out five hundred and fifty pounds, and now I weigh two hundred and seventy-five. It doesn't matter the length of time to get there. Keep at it. I believe that, once you set a goal to do something, you shouldn't let anything or anyone stand in your way from achieving that. You stay the course until you reach your goal. Whatever caused you to become unmotivated will soon pass, so work through it. On the days you are feeling amped up to drive hard in the gym, you feel good that you didn't let that one day stop you from exercising. Remember, this is a lifetime commitment, not a month or a year agreement. You weren't that tired and bothered in your life to eat cakes and cookies, so goes it with exercising. Remember, lose the excuses and the weight. Challenging yourself is telling yourself that you're going to push yourself a little more and more. When you place a challenge for yourself, your aim or goal is to make it toward that point you give yourself. You strive to reach that mark every time you step into the gym. Make it your point to hit that mark or come closer to it every time. Don't let anything stop you from your goal. Of course, you may experience different kinds of negative feelings, but keep the desire to want to be slimmer or get healthier first. Ignore these negative feelings, and spark the fire to beat or conquer your challenge. Once you learn how to think like this, you will see amazing results, and you will feel very confident to take on any task in your life. If you can adopt this train of thought, you can lose the excuses and the weight. Now I have shown you how to challenge yourself. Now it's time to stay at it.

CONSISTENT

Now, THE NUMBER of times you make visits to the gym is entirely up to you, but at least try to go twice a week. I know everybody has different work schedules, but twice a week is minimal. If you have more free time, hit the gym. Make the gym your second home. If you do go more than twice a week, never go a full seven days straight because you will burn yourself out quickly. The human body needs rest and time to recuperate. Even when you have a burning desire to go, don't. Find something else to do that day. You always want this kind of feeling, a burning desire to head to the gym and work out. This aching feeling is great to have, but save it for the days you are scheduled to go. This kind of feeling keeps you wanting and wanting to attend more and more and not quit the gym, and it will keep you consistent because every day offers a new challenge from the last time you worked out.

So once you are consistent in attending the gym every day, this is when you begin to start shedding the weight and toning your body. Being consistent is key to toning and losing the extras. Now, if you want to start developing that physique you have always dreamed of having, you must learn how to place your body under complete stress. I don't recommend doing circuit training at all. You have to place your body and metabolism under complete stress, and the only way to do this is to stay consistent with your workout for a long length of time, longer than you would if you would circuit train. Find an exercise you like doing, and do it all the time. Don't change the exercise, but only the speed and intensity. This is how you bring your body under total stress, and this is how you will start burning the calories. Doing something for a long length of time forces your body to really work and work very hard. Circuit training doesn't give you this type of length, plus it allows somewhat of a break, a rest pause, from your workout. I believe this break in between changing machines doesn't stress the body hard, and it's harder to try to get back into that groove once you have taken that rest pause. You may do the bike for ten minutes and hop on the elliptical for another ten, but it will not make your muscle work as hard than if you were to continue one exercise for a long length of time. In my opinion, circuit training is a short burst of intensity. In toning and losing weight, it's not doing the exercise itself that is going to make a difference. It's how long you do the exercise. Circuit training doesn't place enough stress on the body to build endurance or stamina.

You must learn how to build a smooth, rhythmic pace on the machine of your choice. If you are just beginning and have never worked out before, in order to start building stamina and endurance, you must give your body a chance to build muscles on the machine. For example, if you are using a stair-climber for the first time, you will be incorporating a lot of leg and back muscles. Your body will fight and wrestle to keep your legs and back moving upwards at all times. If you aren't used to using these muscles to perform this type of strenuous activity, this will cause your heart to work harder and harder, which, if kept up for a long length of time, will cause your body to burn tons of calories, especially if you are a heavyset person. That's why I say you should work out on one machine. Allow your body to build up these muscles and strengthen your cardiovascular system.

Working out one day for five minutes or less will not burn or stress the body enormously to see any major results in the future. You have to bang it to the max . . . hard. You must place a serious challenge on yourself and your body. I have come up with this formula to give you an understanding of what I mean: time multiplied by intensity multiplied by consistent equals promising results. You can't have one without the other. You must use them together in order to gain or see results. Now this isn't a one-day miracle, so please don't expect to work out one day and see major or any kind of tremendous results the following day. It won't happen. To simplify my formula, the longer you work out on one machine with added resistance for a long length of time in a time period, your body will begin to burn calories over the duration of the exercise and help build the muscles you use in your workout.

This fundamental might be the most difficult one yet because we all can attend the gym and do a little adjusting on what we eat, but to keep at it and keep at the same routine in the gym might be a little daunting for some more than others. Now doing something repeatedly might get a little boring. If you want to slim down, you must keep blasting at your workout over and over. It's just like you did when you put on all that weight. You ate over and over and over. The same rules apply when taking it off. Now in order to keep the burning drive and motivation, you must be comfortable while working out, and comfort is key if you expect to keep at your weight loss goals so you don't feel exercising is a hassle to get into. You can't be in pain or in discomfort while trying to work out. Here in this chapter, I will:

- Show and explain ways to keep you consistent in attending the gym
- Help you get past a few types of feeling—pain, sick, tiredness, and boredom—that can kill your drive and motivation in the gym

All these types of feeling will plague you from time to time, especially when you attend the gym a lot and do the same routine every day. Comfort is everything when it comes to exercise, and it's very important. It's hard to try to focus when you are uncomfortable or in pain. Pain and discomfort will only take your mind off your workout and keep you from being focused or in tune to your workout. You must invest in the necessary gym accessories (tools) to make the gym comfortable and relaxing to be in. Once you learn how to rev up the intensity and start reaching into your red zone, you don't want to be in pain or discomfort because of improper footwear or uncomfortable clothing. You don't want anything that is going to distract or discomfort you when you are in or coming near that red zone.

First, I suggest you start with your foundation. Your feet are one part of your body that you will always use, no matter what exercise you do. So you would need to invest in some good pair of tennis shoes that are snug to your feet. You don't want a pair of shoes that are too tight or too loose. Shoes that are too loose or too tight will cause you pain and discomfort, too. Buy a pair that will allow your feet to breathe. A pair of running shoes is best because they are light and flex very easily. A good running shoe that bends very easily helps your foot in its gait cycle and helps you move more easily when you move at high speeds. Newer types of running shoes have great cushioning that give a runner a springy-type resiliency.

Buy a shoe that fits your pronation type. This also makes a big difference in your foot comfort. Check with your local shoe store and find the shoe type that fits your foot's biomechanics. If you don't know, look on the bottom of an old or worn-out pair of tennis shoes to find what areas you wear your shoes in.

The biggest and most important part of comfort comes from the condition and type of shoe you wear. Your foot comfort will play a very huge role in how long and comfortable you are while working out in the gym. For example, consider running in a pair of boots on the treadmill. Sure, anybody can exercise in any kind of shoe he or she wears, but how long will he or she be comfortable working out in a shoe that is not designed for that type of use? Purchase a shoe that fits your type of exercise. For example:

- If you plan to run, buy running shoes.
- If you plan to walk, power walk, or use the stair-climber, walking or running shoes are fine.
- If you plan to weight train, you may want to purchase a training type of shoe. Weight training shoes typically have harder material on the soles of the shoe to remove pressure off the foot.

Walking and running shoes are very similar in design and cushion, but running shoes are more flexible and lighter for foot shock absorption and foot flexing. I love Reeboks. I use them when I work out. I have different pairs of Reeboks for different activities of my daily life. I have a pair for normal casual outings, and I have a pair for working out in. Reebok, in my personal opinion, are reasonably priced, and they make fairly decent shoes. I don't advise you buy a pair of expensive, name-brand shoes to use as your workout shoes. Just find a decent pair that is good for your feet and your wallet.

Another good gym accessory is a sweat rag or headband. If you sweat very heavily, you don't want to have sweat pouring down your face while exercising. This will cause a big distraction.

You don't want to feel stiff or wear any tightly fit clothing while working out. I suggest wearing loose-fit clothing and baggy shorts or low cut sweats, if it is cold. You don't want feel like you're working out in a straitjacket, but your shirt or whatever kind of attire you choose shouldn't be too loose. A shirt that is too loose will be more of a distraction than a benefit to work out in. You will be trying to make adjustments, and this will cause you to lose focus on your workout. Essentially, you want to wear something loose and fitted, but not tight. Don't try to look smaller than what you are or try to impress people around you. You are there for you and not to pose or walk down the runway. You just want to be comfortable while working out. I see many people wearing these thick sweaters or heavy cotton shirts. You must allow your body to properly ventilate when you are really working out hard. I suggest a very thin T-shirt. When you really start sweating hard, you want to help your body vent itself. If you do not allow your body to naturally vent and cool itself down, you can cause your blood pressure to rise because the thick, heavy shirt acts as a thick, insulating blanket. Sweating helps your body to cool faster and circulate your blood better. So wear a light cotton T-shirt or tank top that will allow your body to sweat.

Bottom wear should be limited to just shorts. You want to allow your legs to move freely when you start working out. You don't want to wear something skintight when exercising. I know women like to show off their curves, but skintight anything is a blanket to the body. You want to allow your lower body to move as free as possible so you can easily propel your legs and get a full range of motion.

Being very comfortable and loose will help you stay consistent in the gym and extend the duration of your workout. You don't want to skimp on having these items (tools) for the gym. You don't want to spend a fortune on them, but you don't want to opt out of these necessities when you work out.

Doing something over and over might get a little boring. Boredom will cause you to slack off from attending the gym. It is the number-one feeling that causes some or most to give up. People just get tired of being in the same place, doing the same ol' routine over and over.

Excruciating pain is the number-two reason a person calls it quits. It isn't necessarily the pains from the type of clothing or footwear, but the kind of pain from working out or body pain, for example, muscle aches from using muscles not normally used or a backache from trying to stay upright when running or using the stair-climber. These are the most common reasons that people just fail at their goal in losing weight and getting healthy.

Music, one solution to this problem, is an excellent tool to have when it comes to working out.

- Music takes your mind off your aches and pain in the gym and keeps it on your workout.
- Music soothes you when you are really banging hard at your workout.
- Music keeps the momentum of your workout moving, which will help get you through your workout fairly easily.
- Music is a bandage on a bruised finger.
- Music injects that little bit of acetaminophen in your body to help ease that pain.
- Music kills the boredom when you spend long periods in the gym.

When you are really up there in RPM and your lungs are sucking in every bit of oxygen in the building, you need something to help take your mind off your body and keep it focused on getting to your destination. Music does exactly that. Music helps place your mind in a zone or place that causes you to forget you are in the gym. You don't want to focus on the burning or rapid pounding of your heart from your workout. You want to keep your headphones loud enough to make sure you are drowning out the gym noise and only listening to your music. Music helps you achieve that by not hearing the slamming of weight plates, talking, and playing of music from the gym. You want to mentally get in tune with the music. You want to feel like you are there in concert or in the studio with the artist himself. A fairly decent music player doesn't have to be expensive, but it should be from a very known brand. Off-brand companies that make these music players will not put out good sound quality. Cheap players won't produce high stereo sound quality to drown out the gym racket. When choosing the right type of music player, make sure the treble is high and very clear and the bass is very low and pounds very hard in your ear.

Don't purchase cheap, store-brand headsets. Not only they are low-quality headsets, but they put out low sound quality as well. The music will sound like it is in the distance or give off an echo-type sound. I suggest you choose earbuds for headphones. I use them, too. They are closer to your eardrum than any other type, and they drown out the gym noise better than the others can. You don't want to think you are in the gym. Try to focus on the music and not the workout or time. This will help you get your mind off the pain.

You may need other items when working out in the gym, like towels, headbands, gloves, weight belts, and wrist straps, but don't waste your money on things you aren't going to use or apply to your workout. I suggest you only purchase items you need accordingly, based on the type of exercise you choose. For example, don't buy knee straps if you aren't going to use them.

Staying consistent is the key to melting fat and getting healthy. There is no other way to convert your body into the body you desire if you aren't consistent with your routine. You can do a complete body workout in one day and not see any results if you aren't consistent every day. Despite what diet or changes you make in your life and no matter how hard you bust your ass, you won't see shit if you do not stick with it on a day-to-day basis. No matter what holiday or special occasion it may be, devote yourself and your mind to your workout regimen all the time. Never take any time off your workout regimen because of a special occasion or holiday. If it is Christmas or Thanksgiving, don't stuff your face and say to yourself, "I'll burn it off tomorrow or the next time I go to the gym." That kind of thinking is only an excuse to pig out, and that excuse will cause you to slack off from your new change of eating. If a special holiday comes up and you want to enjoy the holiday food selection, eat the healthy selections. For example, if there is a turkey for Thanksgiving, eat that and have a salad with it. If the selection of desserts is pie, cakes, and ambrosia, choose the ambrosia instead.

You may have to cut out some things all together. Remember, getting healthy and losing the extra gut is an everyday job, not a special occasion. If you can lose the excuses, then you will definitely lose the weight. Staying at your regime will only bring great results. Once you have learned how to stick to it, it becomes easier and easier every day, and you won't realize how fast you are zipping through your workouts in a week. Don't try to penny-pinch when it comes to getting the necessary items you need in the gym to work out with. This is your health, and your health goes a lot farther than a dollar. Of course, you don't have to go all out and purchase a thousand-dollar pair of shoes or the most expensive name-brand item to do the same job a less expensive one can do, but you want to make sure you have decent and fairly quality items that are going to do the job. You may need these items to help keep you comfortable. Just like a mechanic needs the proper tools to complete his job, so do you need the right tools to work out with.

CONCLUSION

I USED THESE THREE fundamentals to shed the excess. You can also do the same thing as well. You must put your mind and body into gear. Lose these negative thoughts of "I can't!" or "I don't know how to!" You didn't have these thoughts when you were packing your mouth with candy and cakes. All these specialty machines, hip-hop dances programs, and videos are something you will not use all day and every day of your lives. My fundamentals on getting healthy and fit are all you need and can be applied at any age and any condition of one's life. You must be the one to make the initiatives to start. This book is no more than a guide to a better and fit life. If you don't take the initiative, this book and others like it will not get you the chiseled, hard, firm body you have dreamed of having. If you are looking for fast results, then toss this book to the trash because it will not bring overnight success. Wherever or whoever you are, if you want to get fit and stay fit, read my book page by page. I didn't get my three basic principles out of some weight loss magazine. I didn't undergo some special studies out of some research center in some foreign country. I didn't get my testimonials from people I received information from. I'm the testimonial. I'm the research rat out of my own home. These three fundamentals are derived from my own experiments and research. My success sure wasn't a one-day trial and error routine. It took years to come up with these three basics on ways to get healthy and fit. Now I want to share my story with you so you won't take the years it took me to get where I am. It isn't as hard as you may think if you put your mind to it. It just takes solid dedication and a little bit of effort. It's not an algebraic equation. It's very simple. You just have to get off your ass and get to work. I believe it just takes a little bit at a time. Once you have taken little bitty steps, you will see big results. Then once you do see these results and have trained yourself how to change what you eat and do, set yourself a goal, and stick with it. Then you have lost the excuses and the weight all in one.

These fundamental steps I have formulated is all you need to begin your new alternative lifestyle to achieve unbelievable results and get the weight and body you have always desired and dreamed of having. These fundamentals have taken me to physical abilities and stamina I've never had in my entire life. I still use these basic steps today, no matter what I'm doing. These fundamentals are no magic wonders, scientific research studies, and new science breakthroughs. It's just years of pure trial and error and a whole lot of experimenting with self. You don't need a four-year degree to know how to use these fundamental steps. You just need a willing soul and an able body with a determined heart. Don't rush it. Start out doing a little at a time. Don't try to hit it hard in just your first few days or months. Little-bitty steps will lead to big gains and amazing results. Remember, you didn't get where you currently are overnight. It took time and years, so, like everything else, including your way toward a new alternative life, it's going to take a while to achieve the weight and body you want. Just focus on building or working on your preset goal or mark you choose and always aim to hit that mark. Once you have reached your mark, set out to climb toward your next preset mark or goal. Once you learn how to conquer your goals and work at completing them with my fundamental steps, the weight will vanish at rapid rates. Once you have mastered your new life, set realistic goals for yourself, goals that aren't too far of defeating or reaching, goals that aren't too extraordinary to reach. This will only lead to early burnouts and disappointment to yourself. Step in the gym to seek to work hard toward your goal every time you step in there.

Now that I have given you the fundamentals on your new alternative life, it's time to get started. Now that you lost the excuses, it's time to lose the weight. I'll see you in the gym . . . TOMORROW!

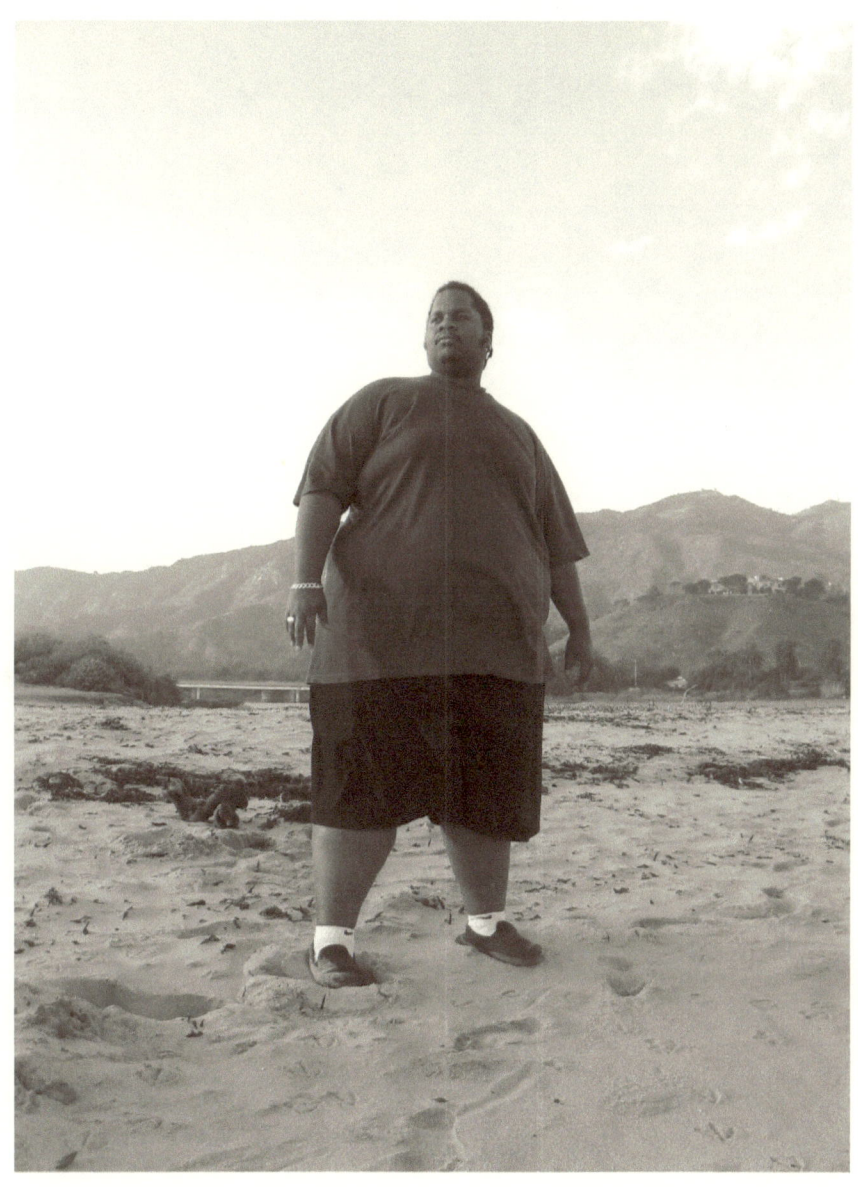

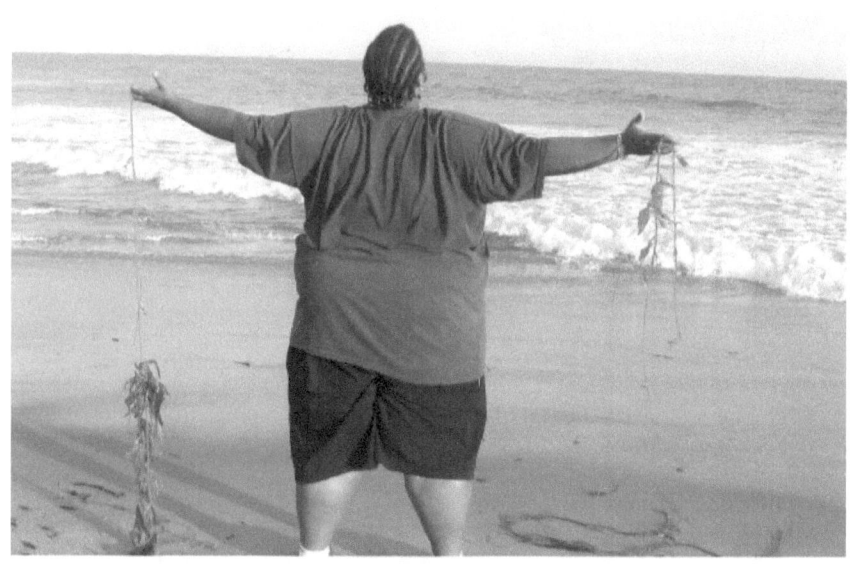

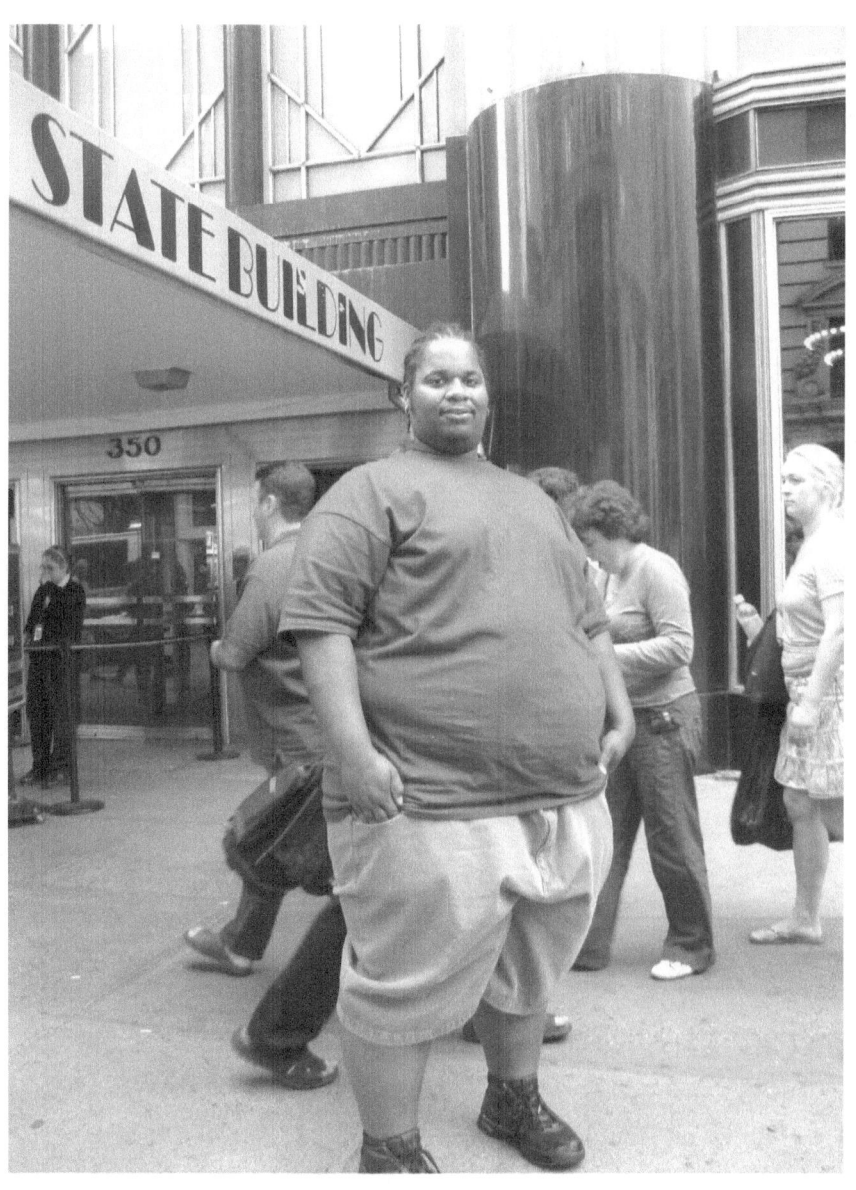

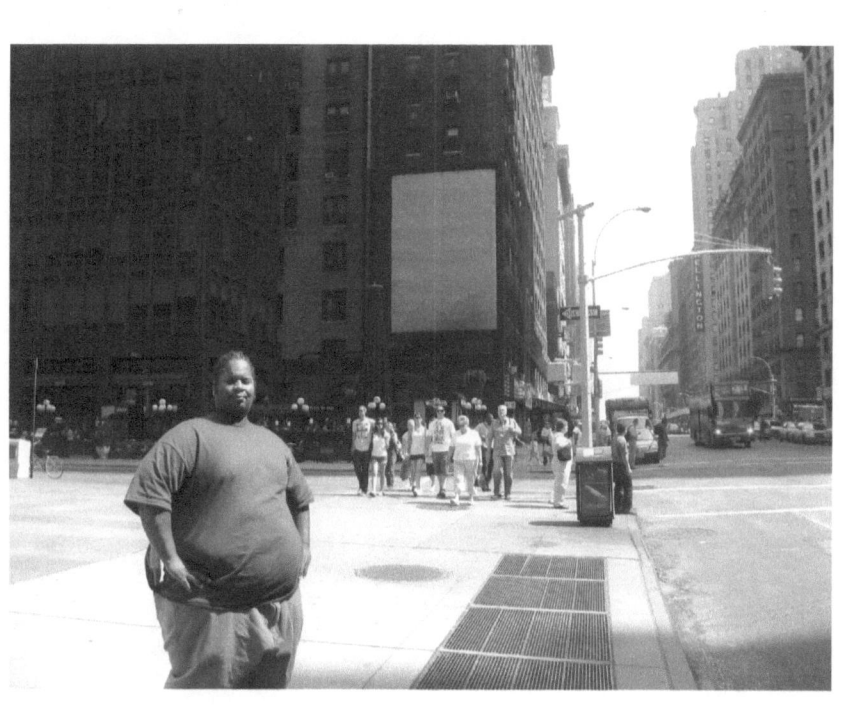

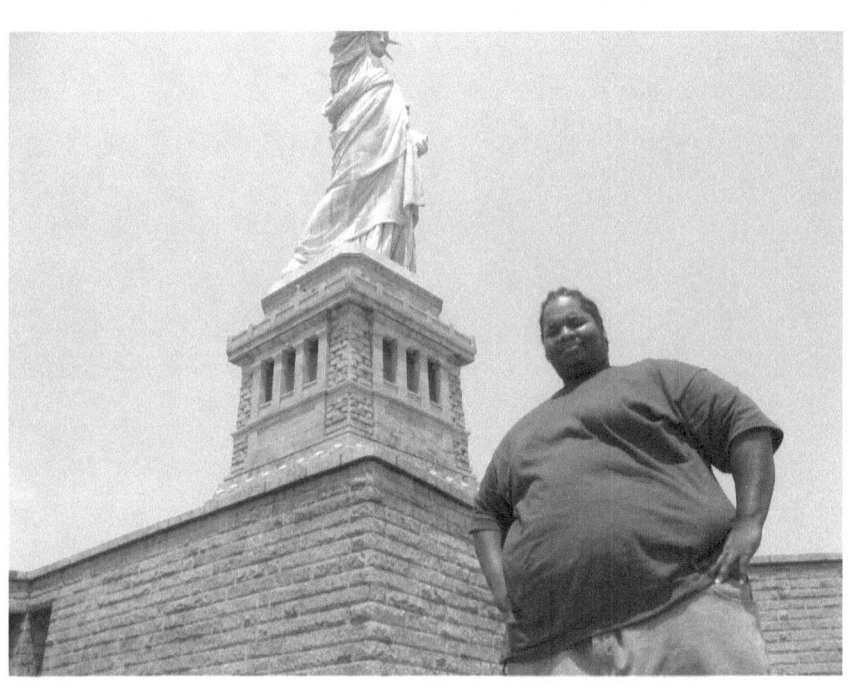

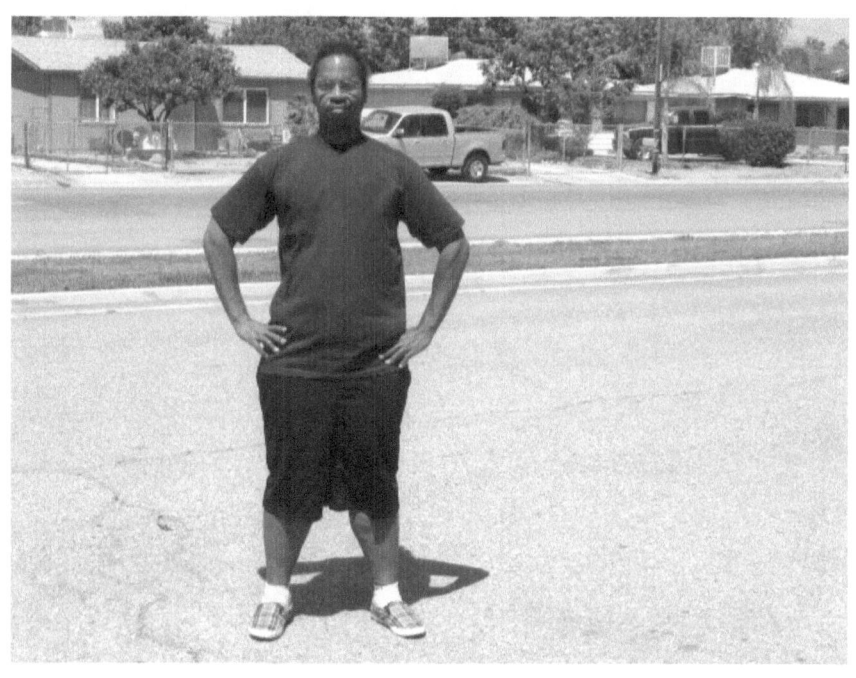

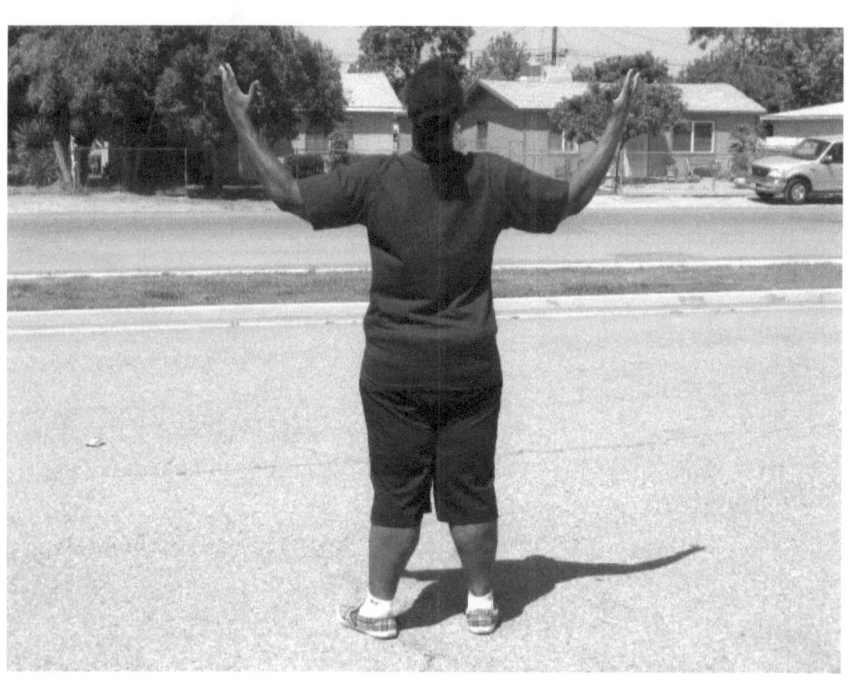

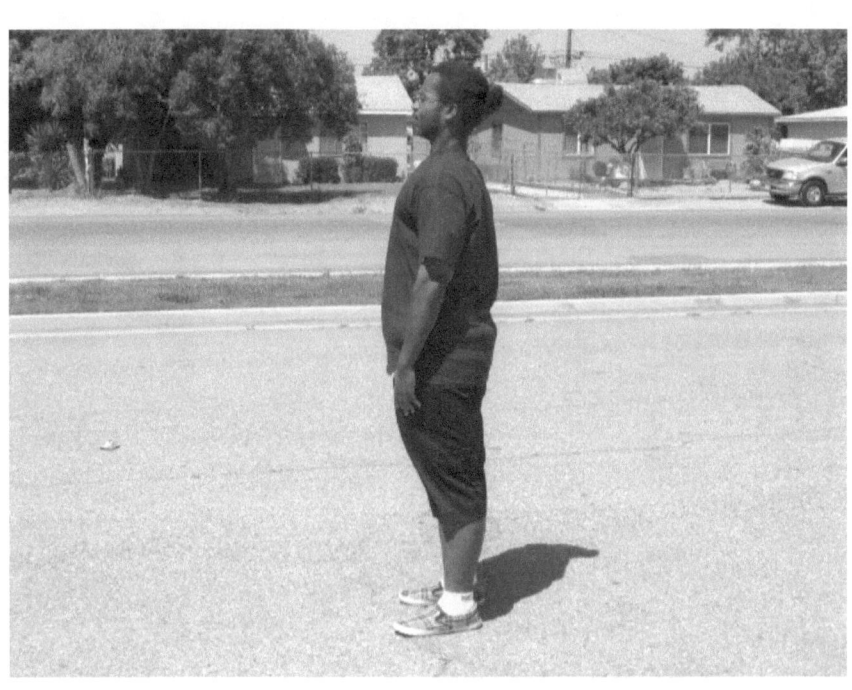

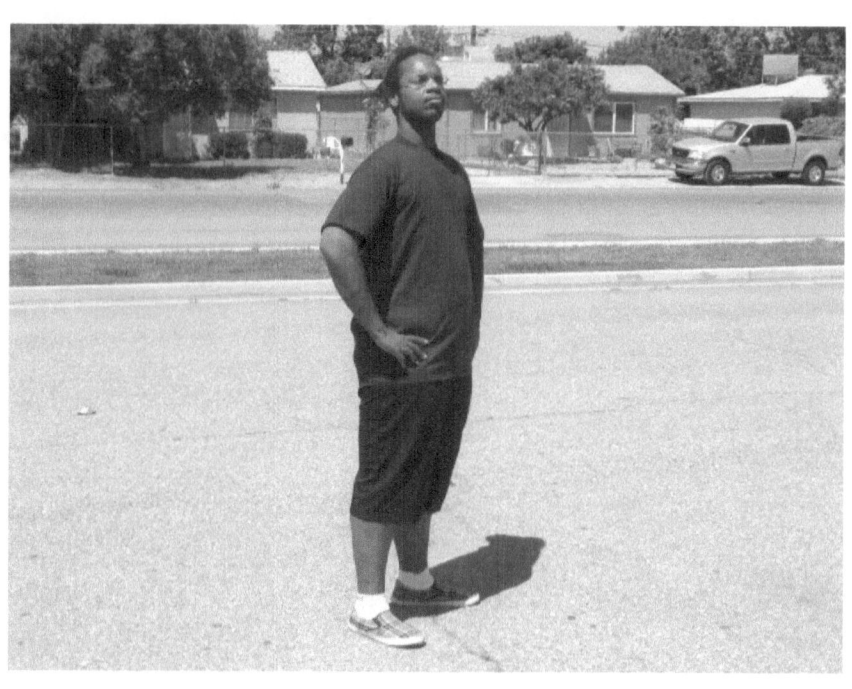

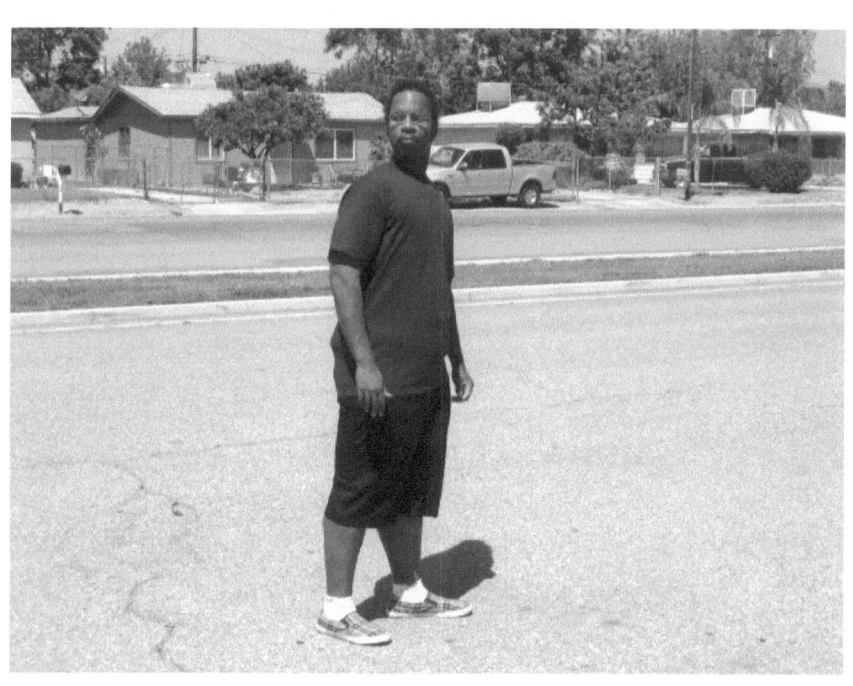